Insider Wine Making Secrets

What the Masters won't tell you...!

**(Everything You Wanted To Know About Wine
But Didn't Know To Ask!)**

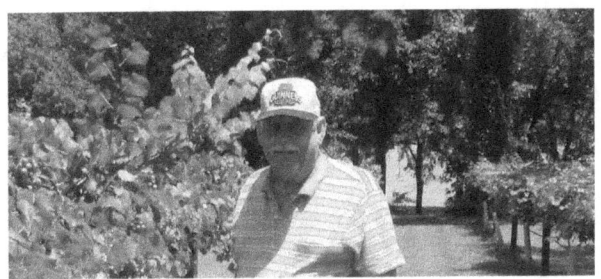

By N. Joe Snow

Copyright 2015

Table of Contents

Preface

I started making wine in the spring of 2007, the year my father died. Dad was raised out in the country on a small farm in Texas. One of his good friends, Chester Johnson, was an African American about 15 years older than Dad. Chester taught Dad how to make wine from the mustang grapes (also known as cutthroat grapes because of their bitterness) that grew wild in the countryside. There are only two uses for those sour grapes, jelly and wine, and the processes to produce them require one heck of a lot of sugar. After learning how to make wine from Chester, Dad made Mustang Wine every year when the grapes were ripe. Dad's wine making evolved into a family tradition. Every Thanksgiving, the whole family, including children and grandchildren, would go to Mom and Dad's house for the feast. There would always be a bottle of Dad's wine for each family to take home. It was bottled in old whiskey and wine bottles which had screw-on caps since the only

—

corks Dad had were for fishing (he was an avid fisherman, but that's another story.)

Dad's wine wasn't very good. The recipe called for about 40% more sugar than was necessary and he aged it in a whiskey barrel which had a charred interior. The resulting wine came out very sweet and a very unappealing brown color. Most of us used it as a cooking wine; few people would drink it. Dad and Chester drank it and were very proud of it. Perhaps it had something to do with their longevity.

Two months after Dad died, the wild grapes were ripe. My son-in-law, my cousin-in-law and I decided that we would keep the family tradition alive in Dad's honor and, after some research, started making grape wine using a vastly different recipe. Much to our amazement, the first batch we made turned out to be very good. Accordingly, we have been making wine every year since. But let me warn you; making wine gets in your blood. What starts out to be an experiment could well turn into a passion. Many of today's wineries were started after the owners make their first five gallons of wine as an experiment. Initially, we made five gallons of mustang grape wine. Today, we make 150 to 200 gallons each year from all sorts of fruits and grains.

We considered going commercial with our expanded hobby but after checking out all the federal and state regulations and expense, we decided it was too much trouble. So, with apologies to Blue Bell Creamery for infringing on their motto, at the Snow Hill Winery, *we drink all we can and give the rest away.*

—

5

Chapter 1
A Brief History of Wine Making

People have been making wine for thousands of years. Where and when it started remains a mystery. There is archaeological evidence of fermented beverages in China dating back to 9000 BC. Most scholars agree that wine making probably began in the Fertile Crescent comprised of Egypt, Phoenicia, Assyria and Mesopotamia around 6000 BC and from there began to spread throughout the known world. Greek, Phoenician and Roman civilizations all made significant contributions to the growth of viticulture. Virtually all of the major wine producing regions of Western Europe were established by the Romans.

Wine has played an important role in many religious ceremonies. The Egyptians associated red wine with blood and it was used by the Greeks and Romans in rituals relevant to their gods. Judaism and Christianity incorporate wine in some ceremonies. From a Biblical point of view, Noah might be considered the father of viticulture (The cultivation of grapes and grapevines) considering the fact that he planted a vineyard after the big flood destroyed the earth (Genesis 9:20). In an ancient Persian legend, King Jamshid is said to have ousted a

—

6

woman from his harem causing her to become suicidal. Going to the King's storehouse, the woman found a jar marked poison which contained grapes which had spoiled. After drinking the fermented wine, she felt much better and her mood improved such that she took some of the liquid to the King. Jamshid enjoyed the drink so much that he welcomed the woman back to his harem and decreed that all the grapes grown in Persepolis be devoted to making wine.

Greek mythology includes the exploits of Dionysus and his discovery of viticulture at the fictional Mount Nysa. It was said that Dionysus taught the people of central Anatolia the practice of farming grapes and making wine. As the last god to be accepted into Mt. Olympus, his reward was to become the god of the grape harvest, winemaking and wine. Dionysus was known by the Romans as the god Bacchus whose wine, music and ecstatic dancing freed his followers from self-conscious fear and care (sounds like a few people I know from New Orleans.)

European grape varieties were introduced to the new world by Spanish conquistadors. Succeeding waves of immigrants imported French, Italian and German grapes. Mexico became the most important wine producer in North America in the sixteenth century to such extent that it began to effect Spanish commercial production. In this regard, the Spanish king halted Mexican wine production and planting of vineyards. In modern times, wine production in the western hemisphere is most notably associated with Argentina, Chile and California where grapes of European origin are common. On the other hand, the native American *muscadine* grape flourishes in the southeastern United States and up through east Texas and Oklahoma. This particular grape has become a major staple for both commercial and non-commercial wine production in the United States.

Chapter 2

The Health Benefits of Wine

In this review of the health benefits of wine, I will attempt to cover what I've learned from a review of a very limited cross section of the available literature and studies on the subject. Secondly, this discussion will be limited to moderate consumption rather than the negative aspects of excessive drinking. By moderate, I mean one five ounce glass of wine per day for women or two for men since women tend to absorb alcohol quicker than men due to a lower body water content which is related to a higher fat content. This differential is further enhanced by dissimilarities in stomach enzymes occurring in women as opposed to men. Also, the term alcohol in this discussion is limited to ethanol, a distilled product of fermented crops, as opposed to poisonous methanol which is derived from synthesized processes.

Egyptians used wine for health purposes as far back as 2200 BC according to ancient writings and Sumerian tablets of the era which listed the medicinal uses for it. These included applications as an antiseptic, digestive aid, and pain killer together with usage to combat lethargy and diarrhea. In some cases, wine was used as a safe alternate for drinking water given the bacteria killing

—

aspects of the alcohol it contained. Ancient tablets included medical recipes for making a number of pharmaceutical compounds based on wine.

A Danish study in 2001 measured the psychological and social behavior of a three group test panel which consisted of one group limited to beer drinking, one to wine and a third, non-alcohol consuming control group. Test results showed that the wine drinkers consistently scored higher on IQ tests than the beer drinkers who performed at less than optimal levels. The World Health Organization classifies alcohol as a class I carcinogen. While research is ongoing without conclusive results with respect to cancer, some studies suggest that moderate wine consumption may actually lower the risk of lung, ovarian and prostate cancers. Moreover, in 2009, three studies indicated that moderate wine consumption may reduce the risk of certain forms of esophageal cancers and the pre-cancerous condition known as *Barrett's Esophagus*. In 1992, Harvard researchers included moderate alcohol usage as one of the "eight proven ways to reduce coronary heart disease."

Other studies have linked moderate alcohol consumption to a lower risk of dementia and Alzheimer's. The anti-bacterial nature of alcohol may reduce the risk of stomach cancer, gastritis, and peptic ulcers. Consumption of red wine in moderation has been shown to increase levels of high density Lipoprotein (HDL) cholesterol which inhibits plaque formation in the arteries. Consider the so-called *French Paradox* where their diets are known to be high in saturated fat given the mainstays of cheese and bread. Coronary heart disease is much lower in France than in America, for example, and it is thought that the higher consumption of red wine is the major contributing factor.

In other studies, researchers have found that consuming red wine in moderation several times a week can help to reduce the risk of heart attack and stroke, as well as cognitive diseases. These studies have shown that taking a glass of red wine while eating a meal containing red meat reduced the build-up of cholesterol in veins and arteries of test subjects.

Significant components of red wines other than alcohol include **resveratrol, piceatannol, polyphenols and flavonoids,** all of which are beneficial to health.

Piceatannol may be considered beneficial with respect to weight loss in that it is known to slow the development of immature fat cells. It also inhibits the late stages of fat cell formation by blocking the insulin processes that promote such growth. Resveratrol, flavonoids and polyphenols are recognized for their anti-inflammatory and antioxidant properties which prevent cell damage and help to slow the aging process.

For those of us focused on caloric intake, a five ounce glass of white wine is 100 calories and 1.18 grams of carbohydrates. On the other hand, a five ounce glass of red wine is 106 calories and 2.51 grams of carbohydrates.

Chapter 3
The Best Wines for Your Health

Suffice it to say that the focus of this chapter is subjective at best and depends on the singular characteristic of the wines one chooses for comparison. In my opinion, resveratrol is the key component given the inherent anti-inflammatory and antioxidant benefits. Furthermore, red wines are the obvious choice for health benefits since resveratrol is derived mostly from the skins and seeds of the grape. In actual production, red wine juice with the grape skins is fermented longer than those of white wines where the skins are removed from the juice early on. Accordingly, I'll focus on this constituent when comparing the grapes chosen for wine making.

Wine scholars point out that grapes from the **pinot noir** family grown in the cool and damp soils of Oregon in America and Burgundy in France, have higher concentrations of resveratrol than grapes from the **cabernet** family which are typically grown in the warmer and dryer soils of California and Bordeaux, France. It seems that when grape vines are attacked by fungi or other grape diseases, the vines tend to produce more resveratrol as a defense mechanism. It is entirely logical that a damp soil would be more likely to foster fungi rather than a more arid environment. One might argue, then, that wine made from the pinot noir family of grapes would offer the most health benefits. End of story. Maybe not!

Enter the grand-daddy of native American grapes, the muscadine. But wait, the environment of the muscadine grapevine is not the cooler, damper setting acclaimed in the preceding paragraph. It seems that the climate of the range of the muscadine grape fosters entirely different vine diseases such as *phylloxera*. Fending off this ravenous disease year after year, the muscadine grape vine has flourished with grapes having some of the highest concentrations of resveratrol known. Indeed, muscadine grapes have as much as six times the concentration of resveratrol of many other varieties. And there's more. *Ellagic acid*, a compound found in some foods, exhibits very strong antioxidant properties and has been shown to be effective in combating some tumors and cancers. Ellagic acid is found in only one grape, namely the muscadine. Ongoing research is exciting. We might soon have some powerful medicines utilizing the healing powers of the red grape and its seeds and vines. It should be noted that there are many varieties of muscadine grapes, not all of which are suitable for the production of wine.

While I'm getting things straight here, there's another misunderstanding I need to address especially as it relates to grapes grown in the southeastern United States. All the grapes flourishing in the wild are not of the muscadine variety. The sweet ones are muscadines; the sour or bitter ones are mustangs.

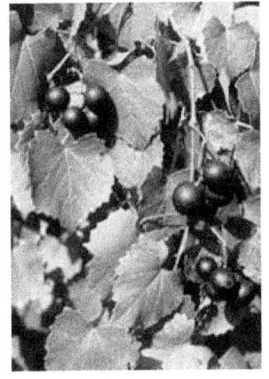
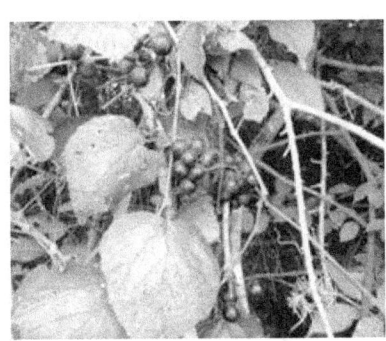

Muscadine   Mustang

Yes, I know they both start with an "M" and that's where the confusion arises. I'll admit they do look alike but the leaves of the vines are quite different. A lot of the old timers confused the two and may have passed on this misinformation to their offspring with unintended consequences.

Given all the preceding discussion in this chapter, my top three grape picks for the health conscious are (drum roll, please):

- Number Three: Cabernet Sauvignon

- Number Two: Pinot Noir

And the winner is:

- Number One: Muscadine.

Chapter 4

Reasons for Making Your Own Wine

Wine has been produced in all corners of the globe for thousands of years but it was not until the late twentieth century that modern technology overcame the messy, time consuming process for making wine at home. In most cases, homemade wines of the era were not very good and certainly lacked the taste appeal of commercial vineyard production. I can certainly testify to that after consuming Dad's homemade mustang wine. If you read the Preface of this book you have already learned why I started making wine. What you may not know is that there are a multitude of benefits you will receive from making your own wine.

Making your own wine is a fun and enjoyable hobby. With the fool-proof technology of safe, low-cost modern equipment and hardware, wine production is a piece of cake. Moreover, it is totally relaxing. Given the relatively minimum effort required from the collection of your choice of fruit or grain to the finished product, the rewards are great. Unlike most hobbies, you get to sample and enjoy the fruits of your efforts. It just doesn't get any better than that!

Wine making is a creative hobby anyone could enjoy regardless of age or physical condition. Besides, what can be more rewarding than to take freshly picked fruit and transform it into something completely new and exciting; something your family and friends will appreciate? You will be amazed at the product you have created. It very well could become a family tradition, just as mine has, with wine recipes and procedures being passed down from one generation to the next.

You will undoubtedly attract new and lasting friends when you make wine. They will want to help you pick or select the fruit and start the wine making process. Naturally, they will expect a bottle or two of the finished product for their efforts which is a small price to pay for their input. And it's always fun when someone asks, "When do you put the alcohol in?" But the best part is when it becomes time to share a bottle of your wine with others. Then they find out how good your wine is and you will likely become a very popular individual . . . you may become a local celebrity. As word gets out that you make wine, people in your area who have fruit trees, grape vines or gardens will offer their fruit from which you can make a new finished product.

Probably the most unique thing about making your own wine is the flexibility it offers. Wine can be produced from hundreds of raw constituents . . . from tomatoes to

---

18

dandelions to rice to prickly pear cactus as well as the normal grapes and berries. About the only limitation is your imagination. You can make two different wines and mix them together to produce a third wine. In reality, that's what the big commercial wineries do. In fact, I've made some wine that I felt "needed a little help." Consequently, I mixed it with a much better wine and the combination was a winner. How about Pearadine wine (a mixture of pear and muscadine wines) or Cherryberry wine (blackberry and cherry wines mixed)? So, maybe you want to be a purist and stick to chardonnays, cabernets, pinots and merlots. It's still fun but it's important to note there are almost endless opportunities.

How much time does all the effort required to make your own wine require? I'm glad you asked that question. You'll likely spend six to eight hours sterilizing your equipment and picking, buying or gathering your fresh fruit and crushing it to obtain the juice. Adding the other initial ingredients takes about 15 minutes. Then, you'll spend about five minutes a day for the next five to seven days maintaining the process. Afterwards, you'll spend about an hour initializing the next process, then an additional hour for the last intermediate step several weeks later prior to bottling which will take less than two hours. Now let's add up the time you've invested. You've probably spent maybe 11 hours over a four month period in making your first batch of wine. It goes without saying that your winemaking hobby will not interfere with fishing, golfing, knitting, sewing or other pastimes.

The fact that you've got your wine in a bottle does not mean it is a finished product. Now, Mother Nature takes over. Depending on what type of wine you're making, it could take from four months to a year or longer to age the wine. Unlike distilled spirits which stop aging when bottled, wine will continue to age in the bottle and the longer a wine ages, the better it gets. The processes and time consumed are essentially the same regardless of whether you're making five gallons or 100 gallons. Naturally, it will take a little longer to extract the juice from the later and to bottle it, but the incremental time invested is marginal.

All right, you've convinced me that I have the time for a wine making hobby, but how much does it cost? Good question. Wine making, like gardening, is one of the least expensive hobbies one could enjoy. The basic cost of the equipment needed to make five gallons of wine will be about $150 or a little less as of this writing (you can spend more, if you wish). You could actually make wine without the recommended equipment but the old adage that **you get what you pay for** certainly applies. From a safety and health viewpoint, you might not want to drink the product.

Compare this figure with the cost of a set of golf clubs or a fishing rod, reel and tackle box. The good news is that the equipment can be used over and over again to make thousands of gallons. You'll probably spend about $25 for the chemicals and other ingredients needed for your first batch exclusive of the fruit. The fruit cost varies from $0 to maybe as much as $100, depending on the source and the fruit chosen. Given that each gallon of wine will yield a little less than five finished bottles, your unit production cost will vary from $1.05 to $5.00 per bottle for a five gallon batch.

Finally, the number one reason for making your own wine is that it will taste better than any wine you can buy from the store. There are a number of reasons why this is true. First, you will control every step of the process and you will taste and sample the product at every stage. Just before bottling, you will make any necessary final adjustments to make the wine taste exactly like you want it. You will learn to make these adjustments later in this book. Commercial wineries make their products according to the tastes of their individual wine masters. Accordingly, there are literally thousands of varieties and versions of commercial wines.

Personally, I have not had commercial wine in a number of years. Recently, I attended a dinner party with more than

50 other guests. As usual, I brought several bottles of my wine as a gift for the host. Thirty minutes or so into the evening, I noticed the wine that I brought was gone with nothing left but the empty bottles. All that remained were commercial wines including a wine I can't recall and a chardonnay. So, I tried the chardonnay and I was amazed that it had no body. I tried the other wine and it, too, had no body. I guess I was so accustomed to my wine that I had forgotten what commercial wines were all about. I can assure you there is no comparison. One more thing I should mention is that you will always have an appropriate gift on hand with your own wine for the person who has everything and you will not have to go shopping for it.

Chapter 5

The Winemaking Process
and Equipment Needed

Making wine is not rocket science. It could be argued that there is as much art as there is science in the process. The truth of the matter is that anyone with a good recipe can make good wine at home. There are a multitude of ways to make wine and not all of them are good. Recently, a friend from the West Coast came to visit me. When he saw the equipment I use in my little home winery, he commented that he makes wine without all the fancy equipment. So I asked him to define his process. He confided that he buys several large bunches of concord grapes and mashes them up. Then, he adds water and covers up the pot and lets it sit for a few months. Then he scrapes off all the mold and crud. The remaining liquid is his finished product which he pronounced "pretty good." I'm not sure if he really came from the West Coast or another planet. When I use the term good, I mean your homemade wine will probably be better than anything you can purchase at the store.

You should be very careful when accepting advice on how to make wine. The Internet is loaded with questionable processes. I'll give you a couple of examples of what I'm referring to for the sake of safety and health. First, you should never use an old water cooler plastic bottle as your wine fermenter. They are <u>not</u> made from High Density Polyethylene (HDPE) food quality plastics and fermentation can actually release a number of carcinogens which were used in the manufacturing process. It's best to use stainless steel, glass or wooden vessels. If you do choose plastic, just make sure it's food grade and suitable for wine making. Secondly, any number of people suggest the use of Mason Jars with the lids firmly tightened. This is okay for the old time Kentucky moonshiner since fermentation ceases with the distillation process. Not so with wine since fermentation continues, the lids buckle and the jars leak leaving a mess to clean. That's probably a good thing since the pressure is released before the jars can explode. This is definitely not the process I recommend.

As mentioned earlier, there are many ways to make wine. To be sure, making wine is subjective. Most fruits contain sugar and yeast. While it is common knowledge that sugar is a carbohydrate, few of us understand that yeast is a fungus. In fermentation, yeast converts carbohydrates to alcohol and carbon dioxide. Simple, right? Well, not exactly. Just because the basic ingredients necessary to produce wine occur naturally, it does not follow that a good wine will automatically result. Good wines require specialized yeasts and other ingredients in addition to specialized procedures. Adding water to fruit and putting it in a covered container for several months will not result in an acceptable, much less good, finished product. Exit the Mason jar. There are those who suggest that the addition of sugar, water and baker's yeast to the fruit will produce a fair wine. Like my Dad's wine, you probably would not want to drink it. Bathtub, prison, redneck and a myriad of other catchy names for homemade wines camouflage the end product; they just do not measure up to what most of us would call a good wine. Why? Because none of the processes and the recipes used to produce them are appropriate for a successful end result.

The correct procedure for making a good wine requires good, fresh fruit, sterilized containers, specific chemicals for the recipe, wine yeast, sugar and water free from odor and taste issues in addition to the desire to make the very best wine possible. After thousands of years, the art and science of wine making has advanced to the point that if you are able to follow a recipe and the proper procedure, you can produce a really good quality wine of which you can be justly proud.

Okay, you've decided to try wine making on your own. I suggest you start with making five or six gallons. If you start with just one gallon and it turns out good, which I can almost guarantee if you follow my suggestions, the yield will be four or five bottles of finished product. After sharing with friends and neighbors, you'll probably wind up with only one or two bottles for yourself. This has been my personal experience. The demand for my wine has grown every year and I now make 150 to 200 gallons each season just so my wife and I can enjoy a reasonable supply for ourselves. We have a whole lot of family and friends that like our wine and the price is right! Remember our motto? *We drink all we can and give the rest away*! You'll need some practical wine making equipment to make five or six gallons of a quality wine. Here is a list of the minimum recommended paraphernalia:

- One five or six gallon glass or certified food grade quality plastic carboy (jug).
- One eight to ten gallon certified food grade plastic tub with lid.
- Two straining bags with draw strings.
- One or two "S" shaped air locks with rubber carboy bungs.
- A hydrometer that measures specific gravity, brix (percent sugar), and potential percent alcohol.
- A test jar to hold the hydrometer and wine for testing.
- Siphoning tube with cut-off for racking wine from one container to another and for bottling.

- Acid test kit.

This should be an initial investment of 75 – 100 dollars.

There are other items that you'll want to consider after you've convinced yourself that you really can make a decent wine and they might add an additional cost of maybe as much as fifty dollars:

- Stirring device for an electric drill
- Corks
- Corking apparatus
- Carboy cleaning brush
- Carboy handle
- One gallon glass jug with an airlock and a bung to fit.

Now remember, the equipment listed above is an initial investment. You'll be able to use it over and over again making thousands of gallons of wine, unless, of course, you break something. A number of commercially available equipment packages are listed in the Appendix.

The following list of chemicals which should cost about 25 dollars, on the other hand, are a recurring incremental cost, and will need to be replaced as they are consumed:

- *Acid Blend* which is used in wines to help balance the three main acids in a wine. Balancing the acidity makes it easier for the yeast to ferment properly. Acid blend is made up of 50% malic acid, 40% citric acid and 10% tartaric acid.
- *Tartaric Acid*, one teaspoon of which will increase the acidity of the wine by 0.1% per gallon.
- *Citric Acid* which can be used in sanitizing solutions and to lower the pH.
- *Potassium Bicarbonate* which is used to reduce the acidity of the wine. 3.4 grams of this chemical per gallon of wine will lower the acidity by 0.1%. Do not reduce the acidity of the wine by more than 0.3 to 0.4%.
- *Potassium Sorbate* is a wine stabilizer as it prevents yeast from fermenting. This is used before bottling.
- *Pectic Enzyme*, a blend of pectinase and hemicelluloses, contributes to the macerating action on the grape cell wall. This releases the polyphenols and tannin bound polysaccharides.

- *Nutrient* which provides nourishment for your yeast so that is stays healthy throughout the fermentation process.

- *Calcium Carbonate* which is used to reduce the acidity in wine. 2.5 grams per gallon of wine will lower the acidity approximately 0.1%. Remember, do not adjust your wine more than 0.3 to 0.4%.

- *CampdenTablets* or *Potassium Metabisulfite (KMS)* prevents wild yeast, bacteria growth and oxidation in your wine.

- *Sodium Metabisulfite* works well as a sanitizer for your wine making equipment. It is mixed at a rate of two ounces to one gallon of water. It is also re-usable, just sterilize your gear and equipment and return it to the container. I use a one gallon glass jug with a screw-on cap.

You will not use all of these chemicals for every batch of wine you produce. The actual chemicals needed depend on the fruit you choose as the basis for your wine. There are different recipes for different fruits and the chemicals vary based on these recipes. Initially, you should only buy the chemicals spelled out in your recipe.

In summary, you can get started in your home wine making hobby with an initial investment of less than

$150.00. Like golf clubs or fishing tackle, however, you can spend much more. As I said early on in this book, a large number of present day commercial wineries in this country evolved from an initial experiment making five or six gallons of wine.

Now, let's examine the incremental basic cost of making grape wine at home. At today's market price of grapes of about $2.15 per pound and assuming six pounds per gallon in a typical recipe, the cost for the fruit would be about $78.00. Sugar at $.55 per pound and two pounds per gallon would be about $7.00. Yeast at $1.00 and chemicals including nutrient about $4.00 for a six gallon batch would bring the total to about $90.00. With a yield of 29 bottles (750ml) for a six gallon batch, the cost per bottle would be a little less than $3.10. In practice, you might have zero cost for fruit if you pick the grapes from the wild or if it is given to you by a friend or neighbor. Additional incremental costs would include the purchase of wine bottles, heat shrink caps to go over the corks, and labels if you want your wine to look like a Napa Valley product. This would likely add about $3.00 per unit to your cost. So, your wine dressed in fancy clothes costs you a little more than $6.00 per bottle. Compare this number with the price of a decent wine in your market or liquor store. I actually save about $1.00 per bottle by going to local commercial wineries and asking them to save the bottles from their wine tasting sessions for me which they gladly do. I pick them up on a regular schedule so they don't become a storage problem for the winery. I remove the labels, thoroughly wash them and then sterilize them in my kitchen dishwasher.

I'll confess I considered going commercial with my hobby but after looking at the additional investment I would have to make to satisfy legal requirements, I decided otherwise. I don't want to make a blanket statement concerning laws regulating wine making in your area. Given that I am in Texas, I am allowed to make 100 gallons per year for personal use. If married, you are allowed to produce 200 gallons. However, I certainly don't recommend you and your wife drink that much wine. On an individual basis, 100 gallons produces 500 bottles. That's 1.37 bottles per day! Hic! That's not exactly what the doctor ordered.

Chapter 6

Step By Step Instructions for Making Homemade Wine

The preceding chapters have covered everything you ever wanted to know about wine making and then some. Now, we'll delve into the meat of this book . . . *how you can make a good wine at home.* As you'll learn, a good wine is not hard to make if you're armed with the proper equipment and you're capable of reading and following a good recipe.

Ready to give it a shot? Good! For your first batch of homemade wine, I suggest either grapes or blackberries as the fruit choice. Blackberry wine will be easier since you can mash them with your fingers to extract the juice. Grapes have to be stomped or processed in a mechanical press as they are considerably tougher than blackberries. It is very important that you read all the following steps before proceeding so you will be familiar with the entire process. Please follow all the steps described.

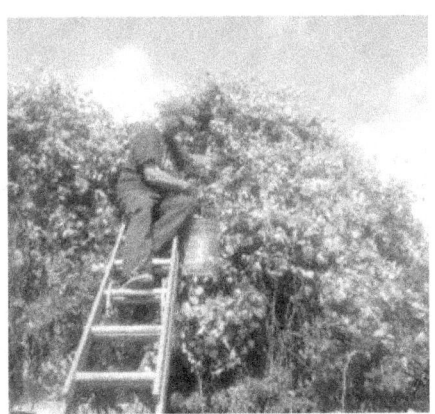

Step 1. *Select your fruit choice and secure a source.* If you are picking the fruit yourself, invite your friends and neighbors to help you. You'll be surprised by the positive responses you'll get. It doesn't make a significant difference whether you pick the fruit fresh or obtain it from a farmer's market of grocery store. Fresh, whole fruit will always be best. Juices will work but the finished product will not be as good. Remember, your goal is to make the best homemade wine possible. Very often you'll come upon an opportunity to buy a good fruit at a bargain price. For example, pears were on my bucket list of fruit choices for wines I'd like to make. A drought in my area had made pears both scarce and expensive. In the late summer, however, a local grocery store had a sale on pears which they had been unable to move at the original price. Happily, I was able to buy the 20 pounds of pears I needed for the five gallon recipe for less than $25.00

which translates into about $1.00 per 750 ml bottle of finished wine.

As an aside, one of the neat things you get to do is to name your wine. Commercial wineries are required to be very specific about their fruit source when labeling wine. Wine made for private consumption has more latitude and you can be very creative with your labeling. In the case of the pear wine I made in the above example, I had about a year to think about it since it takes a minimum of a year to make a good pear wine. In this case, I recalled that it required about two pears per bottle of finished wine. So, I named the wine "Two Pair Wine" and showed a pair of Aces and a pair of Kings on the label and added the explanation that there were "two pears in every bottle."

Two Pair Wine

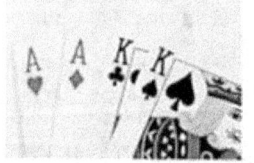

There Are Two pears in Every Bottle
From the award winning
Snow Hill Winery
Vintage 2013
Willis Texas
Best Served Cold

Yes, wine making can be creative and fun!

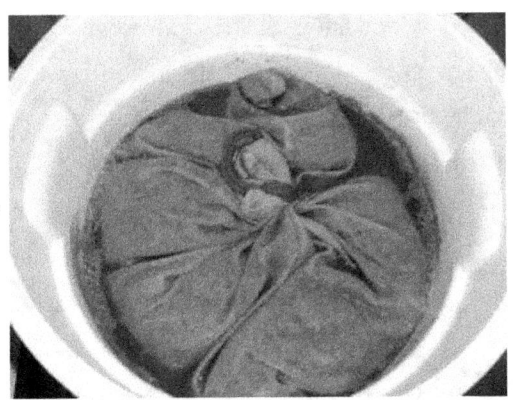

Step 2. _Obtain the fruit, wash it, and sterilize all the wine making equipment._ This is one of the busiest days in the overall process. Start early! Place the washed fruit in a straining bag and secure the opening at the top so that it will not permit the skin contents from mixing with the juice. Stomp or mash the fruit in the straining bags inside the eight – ten gallon food grade certified tub with lid (now called your _primary fermenter_) and add the water required by the recipe. If you are using water from a municipal source, you should boil it to remove the chlorine. Add it to the fermenter once it has cooled. Well water should be okay provided it has a neutral taste. You don't want to introduce a "rotten egg" odor to your efforts. Distilled water would be appropriate, as well. Add all the other ingredients called for in the recipe _with the exception of the wine yeast and stabilizer._ The recipes you'll be using call for Campden Tablets, the purpose of which is to kill any wild yeast and prevent bacteria growth and oxidation in your wine. The mixture is called the "**_must_**." The wine

yeast will be added later at the appropriate time. Now, place the lid on the fermenter and place it where it will remain undisturbed for at least a week at a temperature between 70° - 80° F. The fermenter should be low enough to stir and high enough to siphon the juice out when the primary fermentation is complete. Now, wait for a full 24 hours.

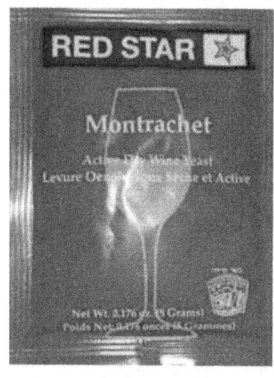 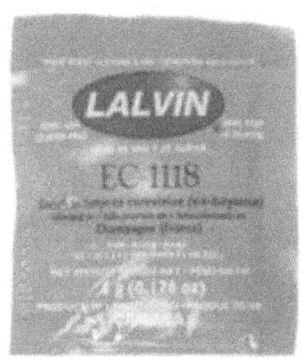

Yeast   or   Yeast

Step 3. _After waiting for 24 hours, follow the directions on the wine yeast package and stir it into the must._ For five gallons of wine, most yeast packages indicate one is sufficient. However, I always use two. Now, you need to stir the must twice a day, every day, for five to seven days. You are now in the middle of the primary fermentation process. At this point you can get as scientific as you wish by recording the data derived using your hydrometer, i.e., the degrees brix, percent alcohol potential and specific gravity. If you're using my recipes, about the only thing you'll need to do is to check the specific gravity of the must each day after day four.

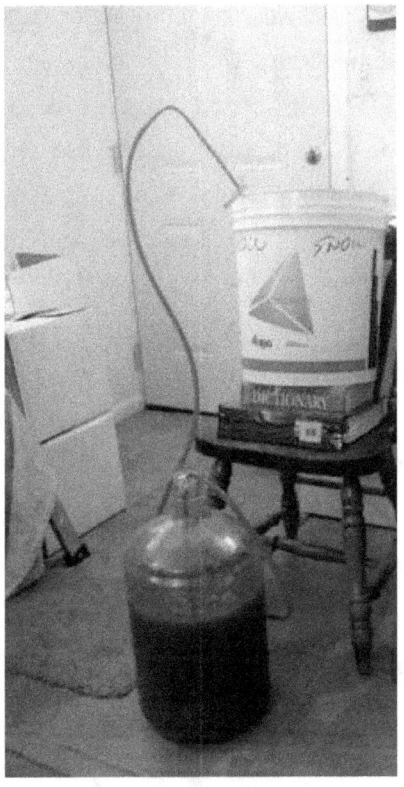

Step 4. *Transfer the must into the carboy.* When the specific gravity of the must reaches the reading given for the specific recipe, usually after three to seven days, gently squeeze the juice out of the straining bags and remove them from the fermenter. With the carboy on the floor and the bottom of the fermenter higher than the top of the carboy, siphon the must into the carboy, filling it just short of the carboy neck. If the must doesn't fill the carboy

to the desired level, simply add water (see **Step 2** for proper water) to make up the difference. Fill your "S" shaped air lock with water. Fit the air lock into the carboy bung and insert the bung with the air lock attached into the carboy neck snugly. You do not want air to get into the carboy. Also, you will want to eliminate light from the carboy, especially for red wine. You may do this by simply wrapping the carboy in a large towel and just let the air lock protrude. You are now in the secondary fermentation process where the yeast is consuming sugar, making alcohol, and emitting carbon dioxide which is generating bubbles. You should taste about a spoonful of the wine, but don't expect much yet since you're far from prime time.

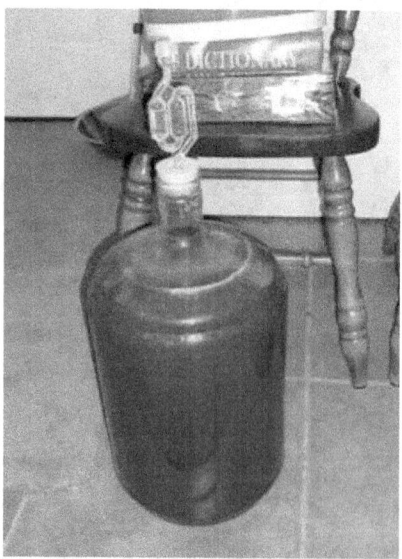

IMPORTANT TIP: Write the date and type of wine on a piece of paper and tape it to the carboy. You will lose track of time, thus the note. There isn't much left to do now except to watch the bubbles which will go on for another two or three weeks, perhaps longer.

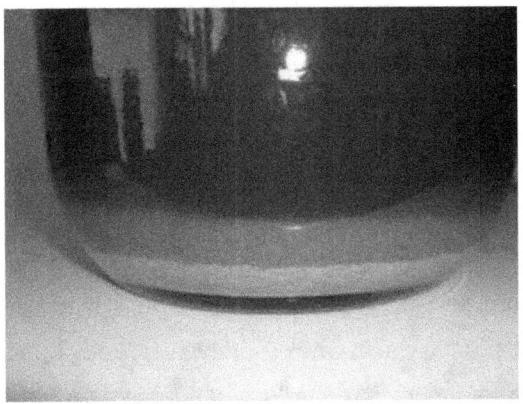

Step 5. *Transfer the wine back to the primary fermenter.*
After a few weeks when the bubbling has slowed to a crawl or ceased altogether, you'll notice a sizeable amount of sediment resting on the bottom of the carboy. It is time to siphon the wine back into your newly sterilized primary fermenter. Making sure not to disturb the sediment, lower your siphon tube into the carboy stopping just above the sediment. I use a clothes pin hooked to the siphon tube which, when placed across the neck opening of the carboy, holds the tube just above the sediment. Siphon the wine into the fermenter being very careful not to disturb the sediment. This would be a good time to taste the wine again. It should taste *a little more* like a finished product. Thoroughly clean out the carboy and sterilize it once more. Then, siphon the wine back into the carboy, add water to fill back to the previous level and reinsert the

air lock. This activity is called racking. Now, you let the wine age for a few more weeks all the while keeping an eye on the sediment forming on the bottom of the carboy. The sediment consists of small particles that the straining bags could not retain and dead yeast.

Step 6. When sediment shows up again about six weeks after *Step 5*, _rack the wine again._ This is a good time to taste the wine again; it should have improved after your last sampling. If very little or no sediment is seen after *Step 5*, you may skip *Step 6*. However, you should check the taste of the wine regardless of a lack of sediment. You will rack your wine a final time in *Step 7*.

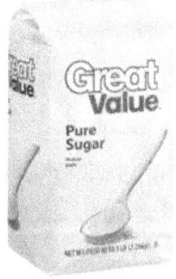
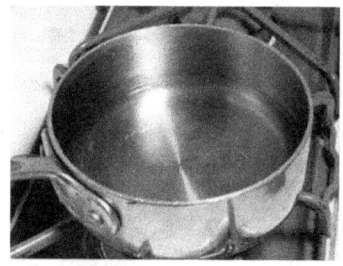

Step 7. _Rack the wine one final time and prepare for bottling._ You have tasted the wine each time you racked it and it has been aging for at least four months. IMPORTANT: Longer is better. You will now taste it once again. How does it taste to you? You are the wine master so you will determine how sweet or how dry (tart) you want the finished product. If you determine the wine needs to

be sweeter, I recommend the following method. Obtain a one gallon glass jug; thoroughly clean and sterilize it. I bought a gallon of an inexpensive wine just for the jug. Of course I drank the wine! Prepare a simple syrup solution by dissolving sugar into boiling water in equal parts. One half cup of sugar dissolved into one half cup of boiling water will result in ¾ cup of simple syrup. Fill the clean jug halfway with wine from the siphon. Add ¾ cup simple syrup and shake the jug. Completely fill the jug with wine. Now, taste it. If it is still too dry, pour half of the contents of the jug into a clean container or pot and record the amount of simple syrup which has been added. Repeat the process adding an additional ¾ cup of simple syrup into the half-filled jug. Once shaken or stirred thoroughly, completely fill the jug from the secondary container, stir, then taste it again. I ordinarily include several members of my family in this adjustment process in order to get a majority opinion. A WORD OF WARNING: Once you've added sugar to the wine, you can't remove it. Please make a note in your wine notebook regarding the specific adjustment you've made for this particular recipe. When the appropriate amount of adjustment sugar has been determined, stir it into the remaining four gallons in the carboy. Let's say it took 1 ½ cups of simple syrup for the test gallon to get it to your preferred taste. Therefore, it would require four times that much, or 6 cups of simple syrup, for the four gallons remaining in the carboy. You'll need to remove an equivalent amount of wine from the carboy before adding back the original test gallon. If there's any room remaining in the carboy after making these adjustments, you can add back some of the wine you've just removed.

Next, before bottling you'll want to add the stabilizer to stop any remaining yeast from fermenting the wine further. Failure to do so can result in the corks popping out of the bottles and making a big mess. In the case of a sparkling wine, the liquid will want to gush out of the bottle when it is opened before you can pour it. If you prefer a dry wine, then just skip the sweetening adjustment. And remember, the longer a wine ages, the mellower it becomes. If you think it needs more time, by all means let it remain in the carboy longer before adding the stabilizer and bottling.

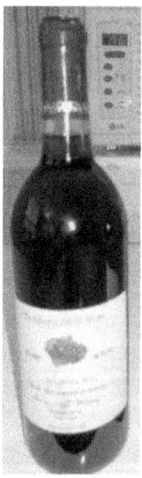

Step 8. _Bottle your wine_. Your wine making process has now taken four months or longer. During this time, you

should have been collecting bottles. The other alternative is to purchase new bottles by the case at about $15.00 for a twelve bottle case. Whether new or used, sterilize these bottles before using. The easiest way is to put them upside down in the dishwasher on the vertical tines protruding upward on the bottom rack. I just put a bottle on every other one, add a detergent to the dispenser and turn it on. The heat of the drying process in most dishwashers will kill any bacteria. Another way would to add the sterilizing solution to each bottle, shake it up and return the liquid to the original container for later use. Rinse the bottles later before filling with wine.

The siphon tube is the primary tool for bottling. The bottom of the carboy must be above the bottle filling operation level. If you made five gallons of wine, you should expect to fill 24 standard 750 ml bottles of finished product; there will most likely be an excess which the wine master can enjoy. Six gallons of wine would produce 29 finished bottles plus the excess. Always plan to bottle the entire contents of the carboy in one continuous operation since air will displace the wine once you began to fill the bottles. Air will degrade the quality of the finished product in a half-full carboy. Accordingly, make sure you have sufficient bottles on hand before you start the process.

I have found it convenient to have on hand a towel, a small funnel, and a pan to set the bottle in while filling to prevent spills on floors or carpeting. When filling the bottles, always leave a little room in the neck of the bottle so that the cork does not touch the wine when inserted. If you are using screw-on caps, leave about an inch of space from the level of the wine to the top of the bottle. Always store your wine in a cool, dark place like a pantry or closet. If you have the cases that new bottle came in, store your wine in them and close the top of the cases. Technically, red wine should be stored in green bottles to inhibit light from degrading the product. However, if you're storing them in closed cases, the question is moot and a clear bottle will suffice. I use clear bottles to show the beauty of my finished red wines.

Making a professional appearing label is easily accomplished with a computer with word processing capability and a printer. Personally, I use Microsoft Word along with a supply of 3 1/3" by 4" plain shipping labels.

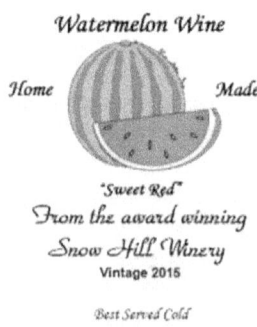

Watermelon Wine

Home   Made

"Sweet Red"
From the award winning
Snow Hill Winery
Vintage 2015

Best Served Cold

The ones I use come six to a sheet. With Word, I divide the page into six equal parts. Applying my imagination, I create a wine label in the first of the six spaces. I make visual adjustments until I'm satisfied with the end result, then copy and paste it into the five remaining spaces. Then, print the labels and stick them on the bottles. Be sure to save the file as you'll probably want to use it as a guide for the next set of labels you'll want to produce. If you don't care about adding fancy labels to your bottles, be sure to add a small stick-on label to each bottle with the date and type of wine you've made. You don't want to be scratching your head wondering what's in that dusty bottle left on the top shelf of the pantry, do you?

There is one more thing you can do to complete the professional look. Wine making equipment supply stores have plastic shrink wrap caps which fit over the neck of the corked bottle. They come in various colors. Just slide it into place on the bottle and use a heat gun to shrink it. Or, as a last resort, heat a pan of water on the stove to boiling; it must be deep enough to cover the entire plastic cap. Hold the cap in place with your index finger and insert the upside-down bottle into the boiling water removing your finger at the last moment before complete submergence. Please note, if you use the boiling water method to install these heat shrinkable caps, be sure to add them to the bottles before labeling as the steam from the pan will ruin the ink on your labels or make them wrinkle and that will not make you happy.

After bottling, it is recommended that you store the wine upside down, or at least pointed downward, so the wine is in contact with the cork to assist in the aging process. This will also keep the cork moist.

So, there you have it! Congratulations on making your first batch of wine. See, I told you it would be easy to make a good wine at home!

Chapter 7

A Selection of Recipes

to Get You Started

Using the steps described in the previous chapter, follow one of the following tried and trusted recipes to make an excellent, enjoyable wine:

How to make five gallons of Mustang, Muscadine, Concord, or almost any Grape Red Wine

Ingredients:

30	Lbs.	Grapes
4	Gals.	Water
12	Lbs.	Sugar
2 ½	Tsp.	Pectic Enzyme
5	Tsp.	Nutrient
5		Campden Tablets (Crushed)
2		Packs Wine Yeast
2 ½	Tsp.	Stabilizer

Method:

Wash and remove stems, leaves, vines and badly bruised or moldy grapes. Put nylon straining bag(s) filled with the washed, fresh grapes into the primary fermenter. Crush the grapes to extract the maximum amount of juice from the pulp and skins by stomping or mechanical means. Leave the straining bag(s) in the fermenter. Add water, sugar, and remaining ingredients to the juice. WITH THE EXCEPTION OF THE YEAST AND STABILIZER. Cover the fermenter with towels, cloth or lid to keep dirt and bugs out. After 24 hours, add the yeast. Cover the fermenter again. Stir twice daily and mash the pulp straining bags with a plunger to assist in additional extraction. Repeat this for five to seven days.

After four days, check the *must* with your hydrometer each day. When the specific gravity reaches 1.030, siphon the wine into a five gallon carboy (secondary fermenter) and fill to within 3 inches from the top of the neck. You can use a five gallon white oak wooden barrel if you can find one. Most oak barrels are in the 60 gallon range. You can always add a few white oak wood chips in the primary fermenter to make the wine a little smoother.

NEVER USE A PLASTIC BOTTLED WATER BOTTLE SINCE THE WINE MAKING PROCESS WILL EXTRACT CARCINOGENIC MATERIALS FROM IT WHICH CAN CAUSE CANCER.

Attach the air lock. As fermentation continues, carbon dioxide will bubble up through the water in the air lock. Keep a couple of towels wrapped around the carboy to keep the light out. Also, the carboy should be placed in an area where the temperature does not exceed 78° F. Fermenting should be complete in about three to four weeks. Syphon (rack) the wine back into your primary fermenter which should have been cleaned and sterilized after initial use. Clean and sterilize the carboy and siphon the liquid from the primary fermenter back into the carboy. Top off the sediment free liquid with water. Reattach the air lock and rewrap with towels. Rack the wine again in three months. If necessary, rack the wine once more just before bottling, adjust the sweetness of the wine if required and remember to add the stabilizer as the last step before bottling.

How to make five gallons of Blackberry Wine

Ingredients:

20	Lbs.	Blackberries
4	Gals.	Water
12	Lbs.	Sugar
2 ½	Tsp.	Acid Blend
2 ½	Tsp.	Pectic Enzyme
5	Tsp.	Nutrient
5		Campden Tablets (Crushed)
2		Packs Wine yeast
2 ½	Tsp.	Stabilizer

Method:

Wash and remove stems, leaves, vines and badly bruised or moldy berries. Put nylon straining bag(s) filled with the washed, fresh berries into the primary fermenter. Crush the berries to extract the maximum amount of juice from the pulp and skins by stomping or mechanical means. Leave the straining bag(s) in the fermenter. Add water and sugar to the juice. WITH THE EXCEPTION OF THE YEAST AND STABILIZER, add the remaining ingredients. Cover the fermenter with towels, cloth or lid to keep dirt and bugs out. After 24 hours, add the yeast. Cover the fermenter again. Stir twice daily and mash the pulp straining bags with a plunger to assist in additional extraction. Repeat this for five to seven days.

After three days, check the *must* with your hydrometer each day. When the specific gravity reaches 1.030, siphon the wine into a five gallon carboy (secondary fermenter) and fill to within 3 inches of the bottle neck. Attach the air lock. As fermentation continues, carbon dioxide will bubble up through the water in the air lock. Keep a couple of towels wrapped around the carboy to keep the light out. Also, the carboy should be placed in an area where the temperature does not exceed 78° F. Fermenting should be complete in about three to four weeks. Syphon (rack) the wine back into your primary fermenter which should have been cleaned and sterilized after initial use. Clean and sterilize the carboy and siphon the liquid from the primary fermenter back into the carboy. Top off the sediment free liquid with water. Reattach the air lock and rewrap with towels. Rack the wine again in three months. If necessary, rack the wine once more just before bottling, adjust the sweetness of the wine if required and remember to add the stabilizer as the last step before bottling.

How to make five gallons of Pear Wine

Ingredients:
20 Lbs. Pears
3½ Gals. Water
10 Lbs. Sugar
4½ Tbs. Acid Blend
2½ Tsp. Pectic Enzyme
2½ Lbs. Golden Raisins (Chopped)
1¼ Tsp. Grape Tannin
5 Tsp. Nutrient
5 Campden Tablets (Crushed)
2 Packs Wine Yeast
2 ½ Tsp. Stabilizer

Method:

Wash and remove the stems, core and seeds from the pears. Cut into pieces small enough for your food processor or electric juicer in order to extract the maximum amount of juice. Put the remaining pulp into a properly tied straining bag(s) and add to the primary fermenter along with the juice, water and sugar. WITH THE EXCEPTION OF THE YEAST AND STABILIZER, add the remaining ingredients. Cover the fermenter with towels, cloth or lid to keep dirt and bugs out. After 24 hours, add the yeast. Cover the fermenter again. Stir twice daily and mash the pulp straining bag(s) with a plunger to assist in additional extraction. Repeat this for five to seven days.

After three days, check the *must* with your hydrometer each day. When the specific gravity reaches 1.040, siphon the wine into a five gallon carboy (secondary fermenter) and fill to within 3 inches from the top of the neck. Attach the air lock. As fermentation continues, carbon dioxide will bubble up through the water in the air lock. Keep a couple of towels wrapped around the carboy to keep the light out. Also, the carboy should be placed in an area where the temperature does not exceed 78° F. Fermenting should be complete in about three to four weeks. Syphon (rack) the wine back into your primary fermenter which should have been cleaned and sterilized after initial use. Clean and sterilize the carboy and siphon the liquid from the primary fermenter back into the carboy. Top off the sediment free liquid with water. Reattach the air lock and rewrap with towels. There will be more sediment in making wine from pears as opposed to grapes so you may have to rack the wine more often. Also, it takes about a year of aging before a pear wine becomes really good, but it is definitely worth the wait. Finally, rack the wine just before bottling, adjust the sweetness if desired and remember to add the stabilizer as the last step before bottling.

How to make five gallons of Concord Wine from Juice

I am not a fan of making wine from juice but some of you may not be able to acquire the whole, fresh fruit of your choice. Accordingly, the following recipe will apply:

Ingredients:

2	Gals.	Welch's Concord Grape Juice
3	Gals.	Water
9	Lbs.	Sugar
3	Tbs.	Acid Blend
4	Tbs.	Nutrient
2 ½	Tsp.	Pectic Enzyme
5		Campden Tablets (Crushed)
2		Packs Wine Yeast
2 ½	Tsp.	Stabilizer

Method:

Pour the juice into the primary fermenter. Add all the remaining ingredients except for the yeast and stabilizer. Cover the fermenter with towels, cloth or lid to keep dirt and bugs out. After 24 hours, add the yeast. Stir well and cover the fermenter again. On the third day, start checking the specific gravity of the *must* with your hydrometer daily. When the specific gravity reaches 1.030, it is time to transfer the *must* to your carboy. Please refer to the previous chapter regarding racking the wine. There will be considerably less sediment with this recipe so less racking will be required.

How to make five gallons of White Wine

Making white wine is a little more troublesome and sources for the fruit may be harder to find, depending on your location. Also, very few of you will have a mechanical wine press, de-stemmer or crusher to assist you with the process. As I have admitted, I am not a fan of making wine from juice, but white wine is made commercially with skinless grapes and I doubt many of you will have the patience or persistence to tolerate the tedium of removing each skin from the grapes by hand. Accordingly, for the following recipe I recommend a white grape juice:

Ingredients:
3	Gals.	White Grape Juice (No Preservatives)
1	Gal.	Water
10	Lbs.	Sugar
5	Tsp.	Nutrient
5		Campden Tablets (Crushed)
2		Packs Wine Yeast
2 ½	Tsp.	Stabilizer

Method:

Pour the juice and all remaining ingredients with the exception of the yeast and stabilizer into the primary fermenter. Cover the fermenter with towels, cloth or lid to keep dirt and bugs out. After 24 hours, add the yeast. Stir well and cover the fermenter again. On the third day, start checking the specific gravity of the *must* with your hydrometer daily. When the specific gravity reaches 1.040, it is time to transfer the *must* to your carboy. Please refer to the previous chapter regarding racking the wine. There will be considerably less sediment with this recipe so less racking will be required. For white wines, the ideal temperature for fermentation is 64° F; in no case greater than 70° F.

These are the recipes which come with this book. A couple of points bear repeating. Pay attention to the bubbling activity in the air lock. When the bubbles cease, fermentation is complete. Give your wine time to age and mellow. If preferred, sweeten your wine using the simple syrup method described in the previous chapter then add the stabilizer as the final step prior to bottling.

The total time from start to drinking the finished wine will be four to five months for grape or berry based products and around twelve months for pear wines. Again, always err on the side of longer aging. Most commercial wineries age their wines at least a year and sometimes longer. But for most of us small volume producers, we haven't the patience to wait that long to enjoy the fruits of our labor.

Chapter 8

Wrapping Up

Well, that's about it. You've learned a little history of wine making and how I got into practice. Also, we've explored the dietary and health benefits of moderate wine consumption and the reasons for making a very good wine at home. We've detailed the basic equipment requirements together with the step by step guide to the process for the home vintner. Finally, we've listed five excellent recipes which will allow anyone to make a good, inexpensive wine that will beat the socks off the average commercially available wine.

As I've said earlier, wine making can become more than a hobby; it can become a passion. I started making wine five gallons at a time. The next year, I purchased more equipment and made ten gallon batches. Then, I started experimenting with fruit other than grapes and berries. My wife, family, relatives and friends loved it. As time has gone by, I've managed to accumulate six, five gallon carboys, one 30 gallon fermenter, two 40 gallon fermenters, and a 60 gallon oak barrel. As I started writing this chapter, I am in the primary fermentation stage with 20 gallons or pear wine; in the secondary fermentation stages of five gallons of Loquat wine, ten gallons of plum wine and ten gallons of blackberry wine. I have 120 pounds of mustang grapes in the freezer which will make 20 gallons of wine.

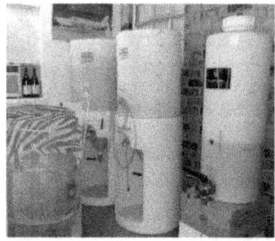 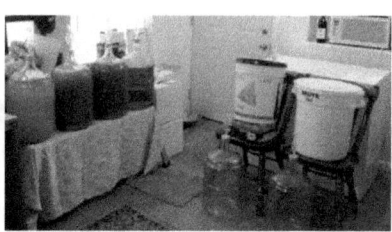

Darn, I just about forgot to tell you that you can freeze some fruit without degrading the quality of the wine produced from it. Blackberries, mustang and muscadine grapes are included in this category.

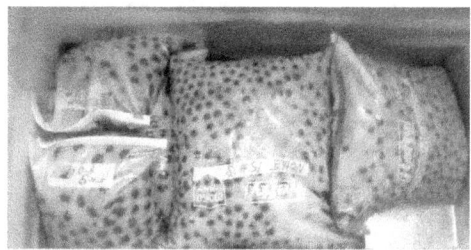

By the way, my passion has led me to invest in my own muscadine grape vineyard. These grapes will be ready in September of this year.

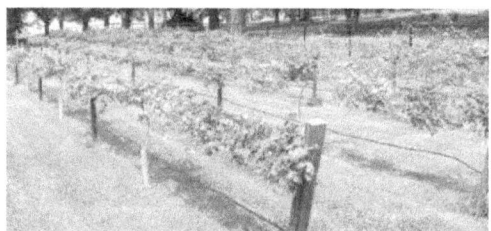

As it turns out, right in the middle of 2011 we experienced a severe drought. I was accustomed to picking and fermenting mustang grapes which grow wild in prolific quantities in this area. However, due to the drought, the wild vines threw off their grapes for lack of water in order to stay alive. Consequently, no wine making grapes were available across a wide geographic area. As a result, I began to search for another source since I did not want to disappoint my wife, family and friends. During my search, I came across an article about muscadine grapes and noted the several varieties suitable of wine production. The more I researched them, the more appealing they became. Now, all I had to do was to find someone with a muscadine vineyard who was willing to sell the grapes. Thanks to the Internet, I was able to locate a lady in Florida who was willing to sell me 240 pounds of Nobel variety muscadine grapes, enough to make 40 gallons of wine. My wife and I made the four day road trip to Florida and back with the grapes contained in two, giant Igloo ice chests.

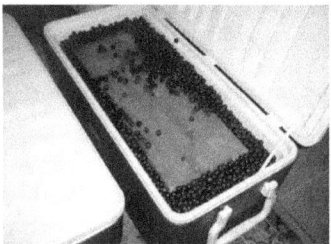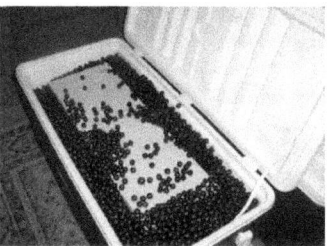

We kept the grapes cool by placing boards on top of the grapes in each chest and topping the boards with dry ice so as not to burn the grapes. Yes, the lady in Florida saved the day but I was reluctant to continue to travel far and wide to find a suitable grape source.

The solution to my dilemma was to raise my own grapes. I choose the Noble, a smallish muscadine grape which grows in nice, tight bunches and the Ison variety which is a larger muscadine which produces looser but larger grape bunches. Both make excellent wines. If any of you have an interest in building your own vineyard, let me know. On second thought, maybe I'll publish another book on vineyard construction.

You may email me with your questions at:

WineMakingSecrets@gmail.com

This is the end of this book and the beginning of your new wonderful wine making adventure! And remember:

"Life is too short to drink bad wine."

Cheers!

Appendix

There are many wine making supply stores. Most of them do not ship supplies to individuals. So you will have to go to them. However, I do have a link to a store that will ship directly to your door, anywhere in the world. Here are some of their starter equipment packages.

This Basic / Starter Home Wine Making Equipment Kit

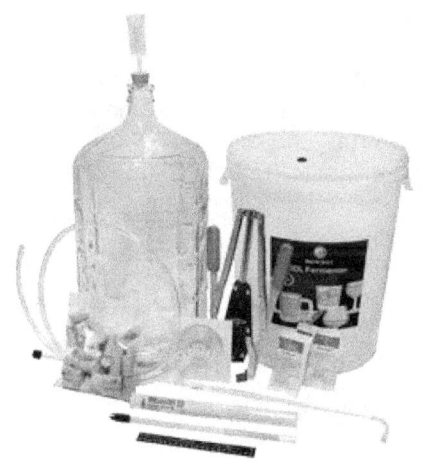

This Basic / Starter Home Wine Making Equipment Kit Contains the Following - GLASS:

- 6 gallon Glass Carboy
- 8 gallon Fermenter with Lid that Accepts Airlock - BIGGER... Unlike a 6.5 Gallon Fermenter When Stirring or Punching Down the Contents Stay in theFermenter
- Portuguese Double Lever Corker - Excellent Quality
- 3/8 Inch Bottle filler with Auto-Shut Off
- Hydrometer - Triple Scale for Beer or Wine
- Adhesive Thermometer for Side of Fermenter
- 3/8 Inch x 30 Inch Racking Cane
- 5 ft of 3/8 Inch Siphon Hosing for transferring the wine
- Siphon Hose Shut Off Clamp
- Drilled Rubber Stopper for Carboy
- Airlock
- 30 Corks
- Starter Supply of Sterilizer
- Instructional DVD

The price for this kit is about $100.00 plus shipping

Basic / Starter Wine Making Equipment Kit - Glass, w/Auto-Siphon

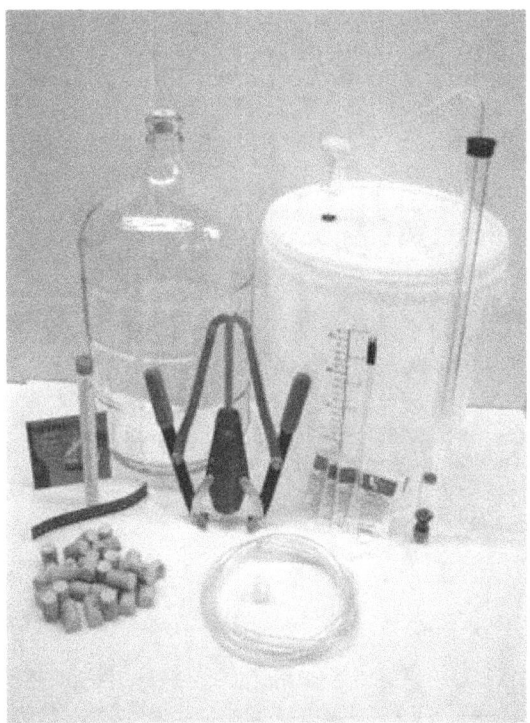

Description
This Basic / Starter Home Wine Making Equipment Kit Contains the Following - GLASS:

(Formerly Called our Vintners Harvest Starter Kit)
- BONUS - Auto-Siphon, 24 Inch ($11.00 Value)
- 6 gallon <u>Glass</u> Carboy
- 8 gallon Fermenter with Lid that Accepts Airlock - BIGGER... Unlike a 6.5 Gallon

---

Fermenter When Stirring or Punching Down
the Contents Stay in the Fermenter
- Portuguese Double Lever Corker - Excellent
  Quality
- 3/8 Inch Bottle filler with Auto-Shut Off
- Hydrometer - Triple Scale for Beer or Wine
- Adhesive Thermometer for Side of
  Fermenter
- 5 ft of 3/8 Inch Siphon Hosing for
  transferring the wine
- Siphon Hose Shut Off Clamp
- Drilled Rubber Stopper for Carboy
- Airlock
- 30 Corks
- Starter Supply of Sterilizer
- Instructional DVD

The price for this kit is $110.00 plus shipping

Deluxe / Beginner's Wine Making Equipment Kit - GLASS

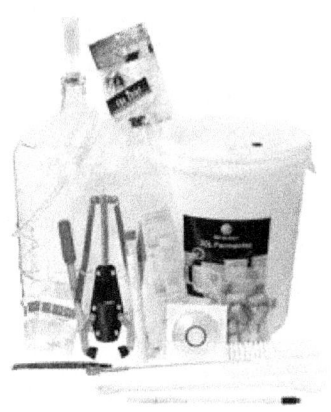

Description
Our Deluxe / Beginner's Home Wine Making Equipment Kit Contains the Following - GLASS:
- 6 gallon <u>Glass</u> Carboy
- 8 gallon Fermenter with Lid that Accepts Airlock - BIGGER... Unlike a 6.5 Gallon Fermenter When Stirring or Punching Down the Contents Stay in the Fermenter
- Portuguese Double Lever Corker - Excellent Quality
- 3/8 Inch Bottle filler with Auto-Shut Off
- Hydrometer - Triple Scale for Wine or Beer
- Adhesive Thermometer for Side of Fermenter

- 5' of 3/8 inch siphon hosing for transferring the wine
- 3/8 Inch Siphon Hose Shut Off Clamp
- Drilled Rubber Stopper for Carboy
- Airlock
- 30 Corks
- Starter Supply of Sterilizer
- Instructional DVD

The Following Included Items are Upgrades or Additions to Our Basic - Starter Kit:

- Auto-Siphon for Racking (Instead of Racking Cane)
- 18 Inch Plastic Mixing Spoon
- Wine Thief / Test Jar Combo
- Bottle Cleaning Brush

The price for this kit is $125.00 plus shipping.

Ultimate / Vintner's Wine Making Equipment Kit – GLASS

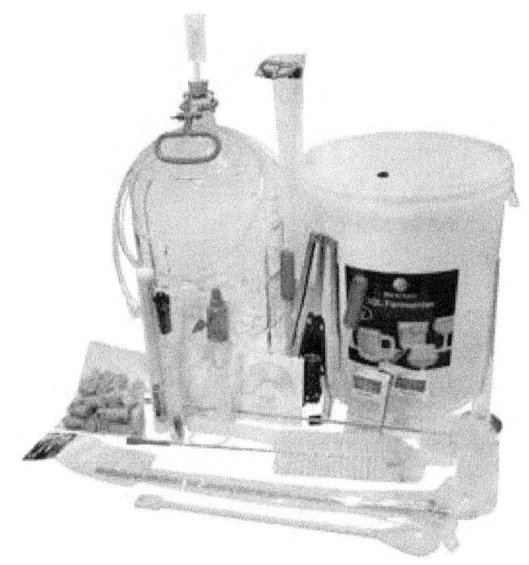

Description
Our Ultimate / Vintner's Home Wine Making Equipment Kit Contains the Following - GLASS:
- 6 gallon <u>Glass</u> Carboy
- 8 gallon Fermenter with Lid that Accepts Airlock - BIGGER... Unlike a 6.5 Gallon Fermenter When Stirring or Punching Down the Contents Stay in the Fermenter
- Portuguese Double Lever Corker - Excellent Quality

67

- Hydrometer - Triple Scale
- 5 Ft of 3/8 Inch Siphon Hosing for Transferring Wine
- 3/8 Inch Siphon Hose Shut Off Clamp
- Drilled Rubber Stopper for Carboy
- Airlock
- 30 Corks
- Starter Supply of Sterilizer
- Instructional DVD

The Following Included Items are Upgrades or Additions to Our Basic - Starter Kit:

- Auto-Siphon (Instead of Racking Cane)
- 18 Inch Plastic Mixing Spoon
- Three Piece 18 Inch Plastic Wine Thief
- Hydrometer Test Jar
- Bottle Cleaning Brush
- Carboy Cleaning Brush
- Floating Thermometer (Instead of Adhesive)
- Metal - Wine Degasser / Mixer
- Carboy Carrying Handle
- Ferrari Italian Bottle Filler (Instead of Rigid Bottle Filler)

The price for this kit is $180.00 plus shipping

If you wish to purchase any of the equipment listed herein, just send an email to:

WineMakingSecrets@gmail.com

for the official link for the company that will ship it to your doorstep.

If any of you have decided that you want to make more than 6 gallons you may email me at:

WineMakingSecrets@gmail.com.

I will give you *special information* which will entitle you to a discounted price of 20 to 30 percent off the retail price if you decide to order one of the following fermenters. Here are the available sizes 8, 15, 25, 40, 98, and 101 gallon.

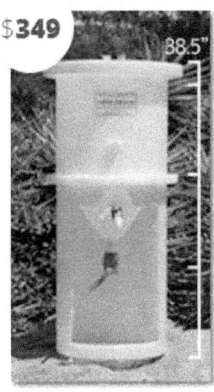

$349

8 Gallon Conical
Fermenter

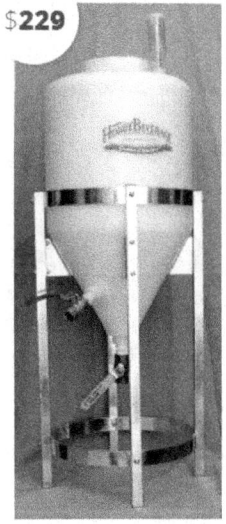

$229

6.5 Gallon Conical
Fermenter

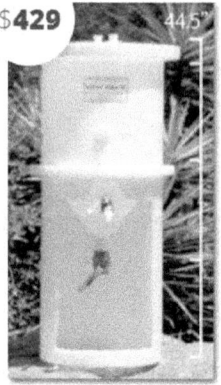

15 Gallon Conical Fermenter

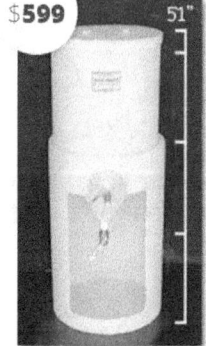

25 Gallon Conical Fermenter

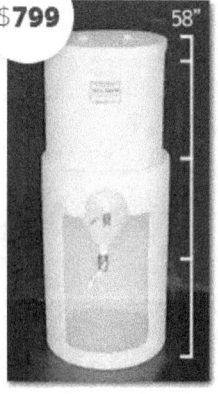

40 Gallon Conical Fermenter

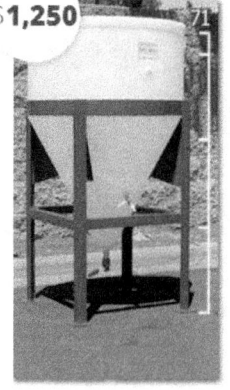

98 Gallon Conical Fermenter

Please note that these are retail prices and were valid as of the summer of 2015 and do not include shipping. World wide shipping is available.

With these fermenters, you don't have to rack the wine. Just transfer the wine into the secondary fermenter when the primary fermentation is complete and wait for secondary fermentation to complete. The reason being, these fermenters are cone shaped at the bottom. There is a one inch valve at the bottom from which you can dump the sediment into a bucket for disposal. There is also a sampling valve above the dump valve so you can keep track of your wines progress. I really love my two 40 gallon fermenters. These fermenters also make it faster and easier to bottle your wine using the valve above the dump valve and they are easy to clean and sanitize.

The recipes in chapter 7 may be multiplied for larger volumes. Multiply everything by 5 for 25 gallons, by 10 for 50 gallons, or by 20 for 100 gallons, etc.

You also may email me with your questions at:

WineMakingSecrets@gmail.com.

www.ingramcontent.com/pod-product-compliance
Lightning Source LLC
Chambersburg PA
CBHW071239280526
45787CB00002B/990